The Art of Training

Tony Kelly

ISBN: 979-8-9868821-0-9

DEDICATION

This book is dedicated to all the people who love to train.

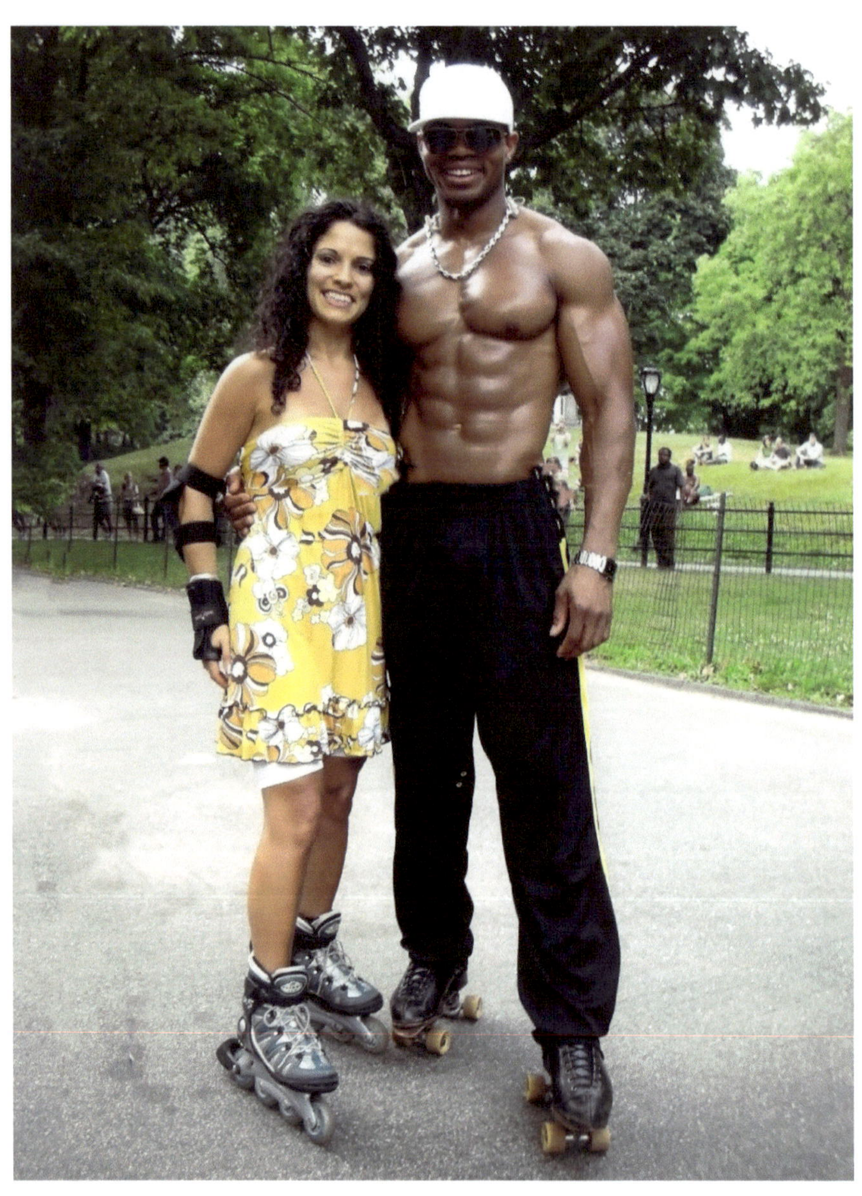

CONTENTS

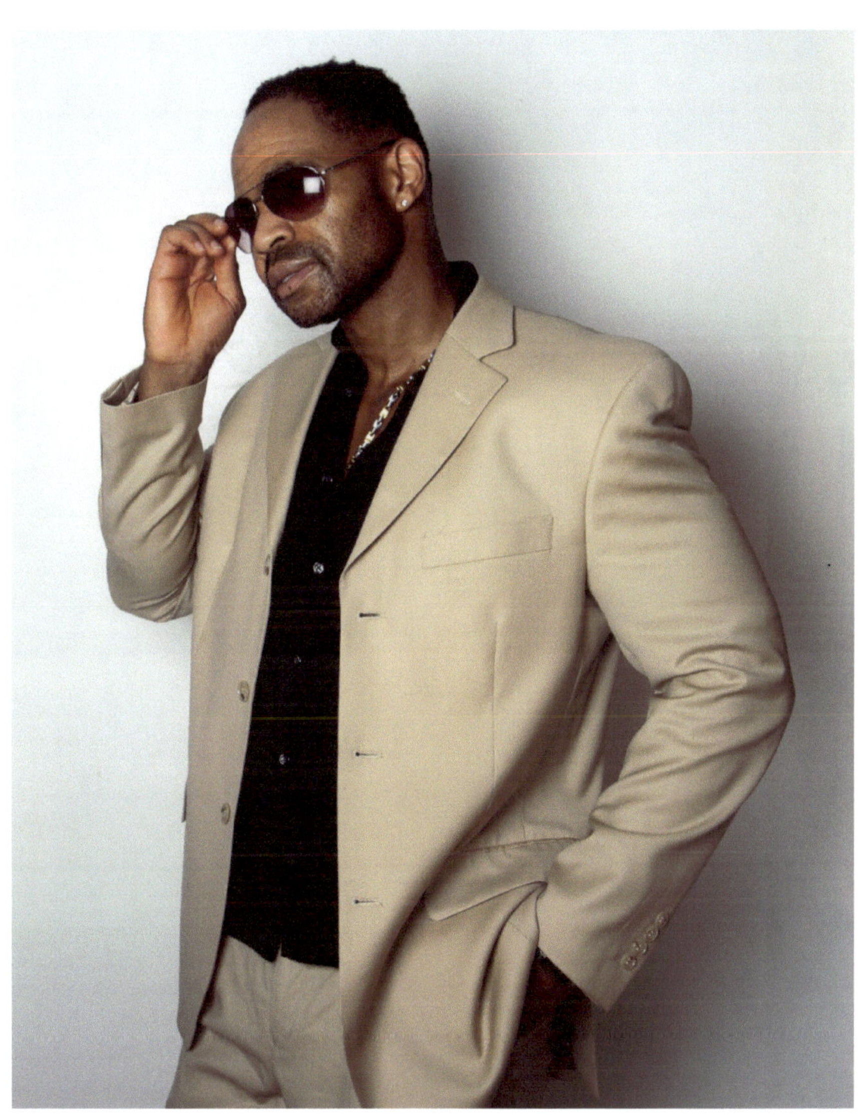

ACKNOWLEDGMENTS

I would like to thank my friends and family and all those who help make this possible.

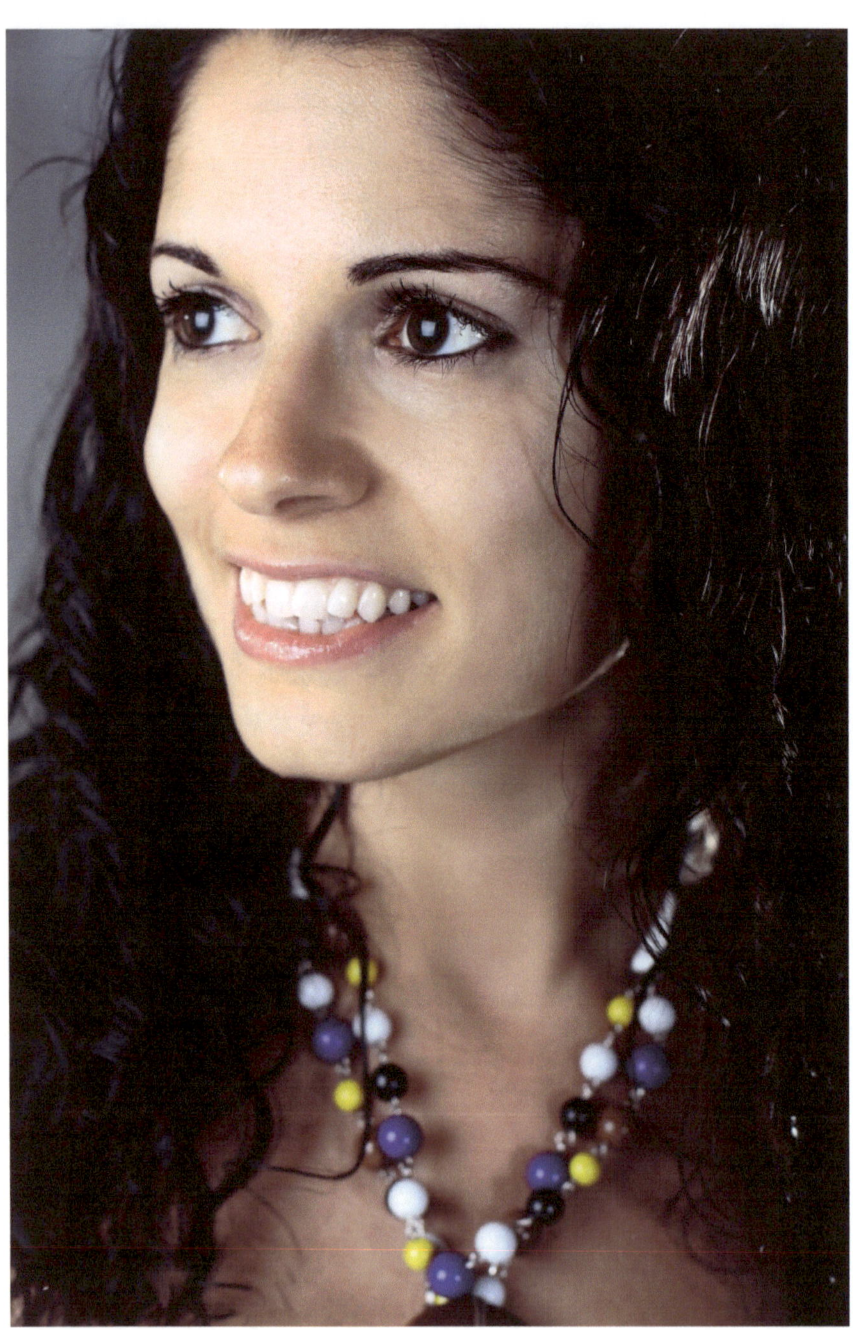

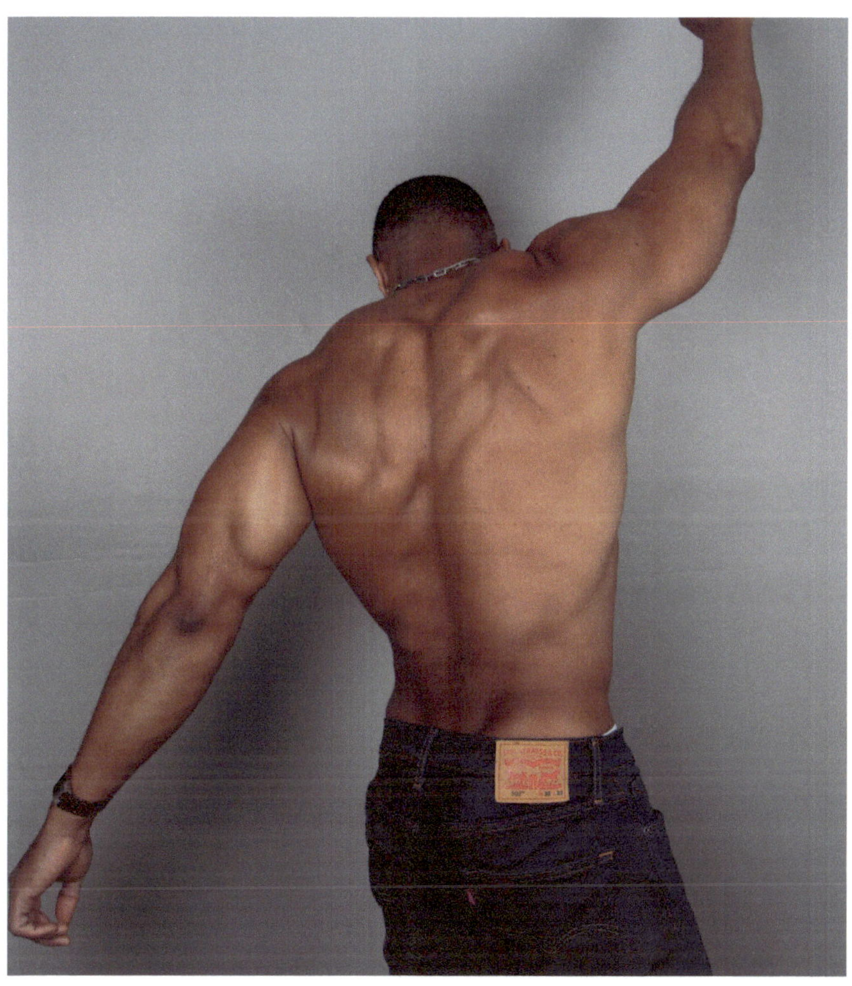

THE ART OF TRAINING

Like a successful Army officer going to war need a strategy so do those who train need training strategy. There must be a goal, preparation and education followed by execution of what is learned.

Goal - Lose weight or Build muscle

An example would be someone who needs to lose weight, tone or build muscle. The lose of weight or toning is the goal or focus.   Next comes study or what type of training is needed to reach those goals. Loss of weight would requires much cardio and possible a change of diet so as to burn more calories that is taken in so the body can then burn the fat away. While this will work great for someone looking to lose weight. It will not necessarily work well for someone trying to build muscle. The person looking to build muscle may not need as much cardio and their diet may possible need to increase in calories.

Execute Plan

In the end both persons must execute the plan to see changes in their body. There is no amount of knowledge that will do what needs to be done for you. We must apply what is learned, this is the same in any arena. The art of training involves Having training goals, learning how to reach those goals and then training.

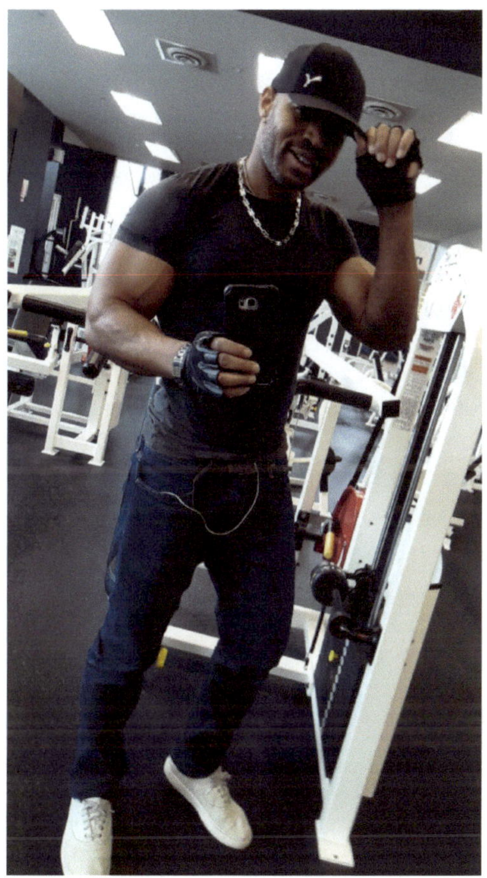

ILLUSIVE TRAINING RESULTS

There are those times that it seems the result for which we train are like the wind that just keeps blowing away or getting further from our reach.

Although there are times when our training results seem illusive, certainly there are times when we can see some progress. Why is it that our training may go without results sometimes

Rest - Seeping

Training results takes more than training alone. The body need to recover from training, it also needs time to grow or change. Rest is a large factor in reaching training goals. This allows the muscles to recover from training and grow. That means sleep should be taken seriously by those who are training for without regular rest result will be difficult to attain.

Eating

 Another factor that can effect our training results is what we eat Our diet will certainly play a large roll in our training results since what we eat directly effect our body.   . When eating supports our training then results can be rapid and consistent.   However Diet that does not complement our training will certainly effect the look of our body as it tries to decide what to do with the extra calories we take in. A calorie deficit diet can also have a bad effect if the training intent is to gain muscle. In both cases results will lack because the food we eat fail to complement the training so the results we hope for will not be possible..

Blind Side - The Illusion of the mind

Our mind is very powerful and sometime blind us so we do not see clearly. For example - A women may not eat or vomit the food she eats because she thinks she is fat where as she is very skinny. The power of the body to create such an illusion with damaging results to us happens also to those who train. There are times that a person training feels there is no results when to all onlookers they look amazing. For this reason before deciding our training is useless or training goals are illusive it is best to consult a good friend, training partner or mate. I do not know the reason why this happens, perhaps its because we see our self often and small changes are not noticed by us. However I notice that when I see people that I have not seen for some time (1 month, 6 month, a year or more) they are usually amazed at my training results. For this reason this is the most dangerous off all since there are results that we our self just cannot see.   The person then change his/her training routine or possible stops training as a result of not seeing the benefits that were there.

    Training results can be encouragement to keep us training. However to see our training results proper rest and eating should complement our training. Make sure we test our feeling of lack of training results with others rather than just relying on our own eyes as we can also be blindsided, failing to see our own progress.

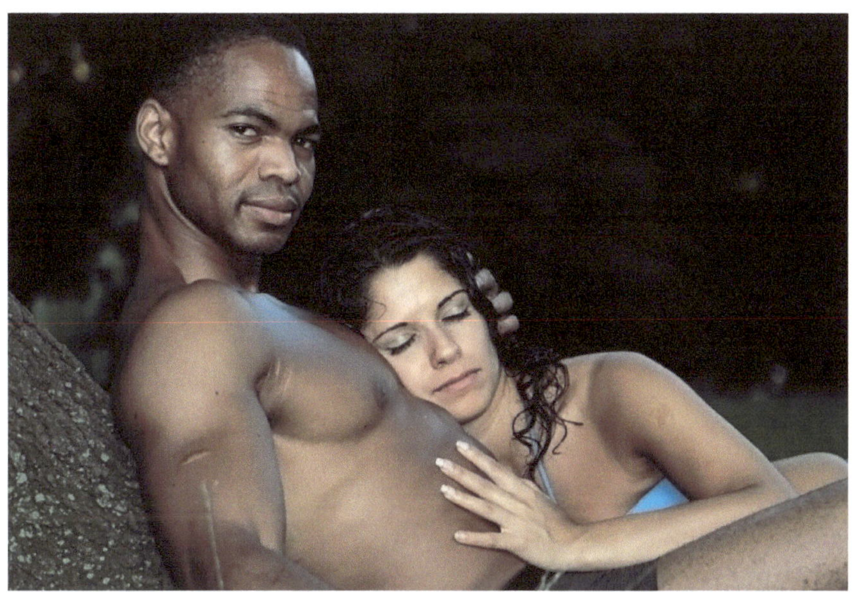

THERE IS NOTHING EITHER GOOD OR BAD BUT THINKING MAKES IT SO

Fitness training is both physical and mental and There are time when physically we just cannot train because of injuries, pain or some physical disability. however sometimes we fail to train because our mind wins over our physical ability.

Although all have different situation in life that makes training difficult a few have proved the sayings above to be true.   I have seen people who look as if they should have good reason not to train training because there thinking did not allow them to stop. However I have heard all the excuses there is to hear as to why training is not possible from others. The difference in many cases is 'Their thinking made it so' , If you think you cannot train with this new job or family obligation or pain then you will not train. However if you think you can train with your new job or family obligation or pain then you will find a way to train.

   Our 'Thinking makes it so', our resolve to train despite our situation is because of how we look at life. When life cannot go on without training then we will make it so and train. When training is optional in life then we will make it so an not train.

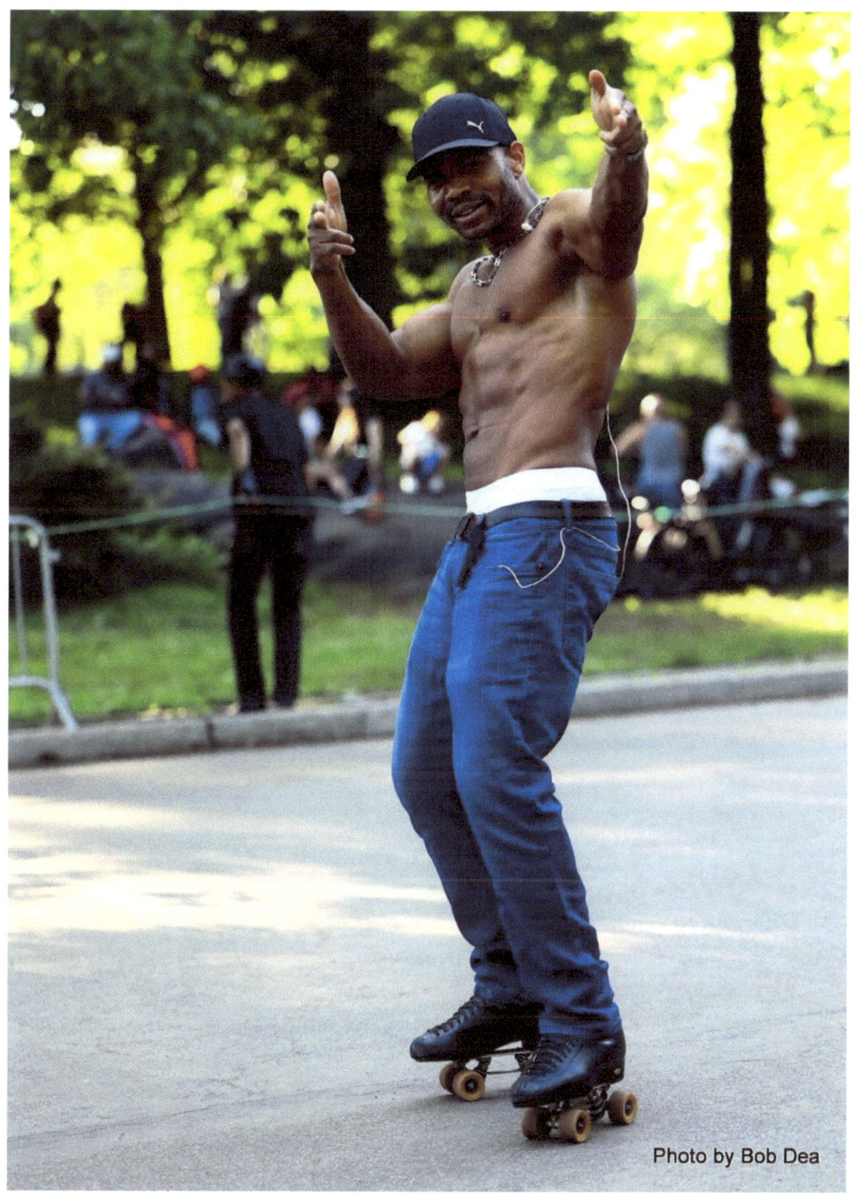

Photo by Bob Dea

YOU WERE BORN FOR THIS

Own it and do what must be done to look the way you wish to look. This is the life you dream of, that of being fit with energy anda body you approve, then this Is the life you should have.

You deserve it

Why should you not have the body you wish to have? why should you not feel healthy and happy? You have the right to be happy, healthy and look the way you should. There is nothing wrong in being your best, looking your best, feeling your best and being healthy. We all have been giving a life with which we can use well and enjoy. A healthy and fit life can extend the life we have been giving even making our life more enjoyable in many ways. This is the life we were handed, it is our responsibility to make it healthy, fit and strong. A healthy and fit body means living linger and happier and this is our right.

Determine to enjoy the life you were giving by keeping it healthy and in good shape. Life will be more fun with a healthy and strong body - take care of the body you were given.

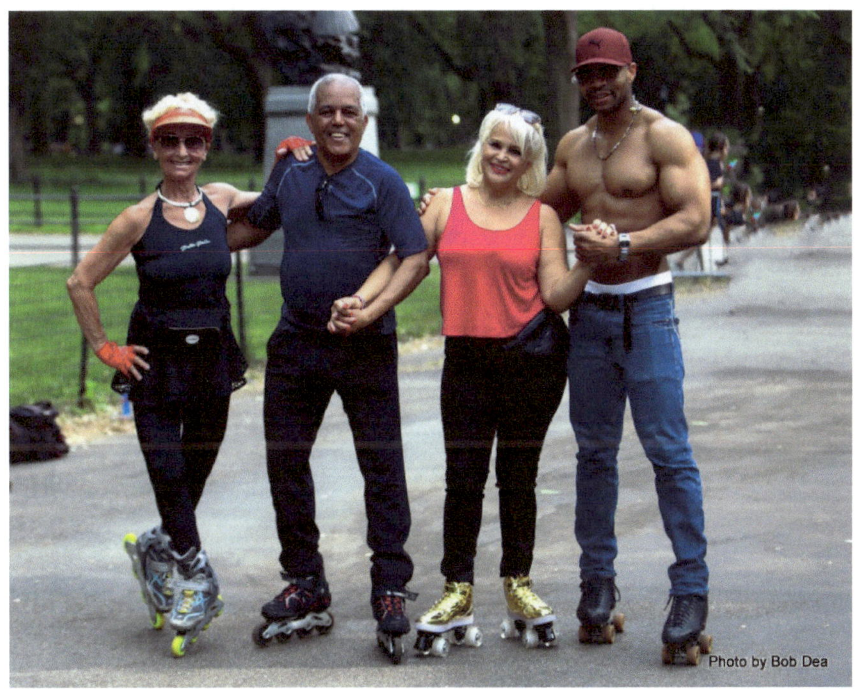

IS FITNESS TRAINING ONLY FOR YOUNG PEOPLE

There are many misconceptions about training and this of curse is one of them. The problem with misconception is that although most are slight distractions others can be deadly lies. Since our health and fitness is directly related to length and quality of our life avoiding lies regarding health and fitness can mean a longer or shorter life.

First of all health and fitness training is for all, true it is a good idea to train from a young age not neglecting our health because then as we grow older we are not left with a host of health related issues.   Additionally if we have been training all our life our body would be in better physically shape as we grow older. However if for some reason we have not been able to train in our youth or did not continue to do so we can all begin to train at any time in our life.

Start slow & be realistic

Anything new will take some time and this is the same thing when it comes to a new physical fitness training routine. The muscles may not be used to it so stretch, warm up and go easy. You may feel you can lift a great deal or there is no need to warm up or lift such little amount. You may remember what you used to lift years ago or even be embarrassed to life such small amount in front of others.

All these are true, you are strong, you can lift more and sometime the training can go quickly when we do not warm up. Lastly lifting heavy weight can be impressive, I myself is always amazed at how much some people can lift in the gym. I am not saying not to do what you can do - only give yourself the time to get there again.

Many body builder who lift daily warm up with a lighter weight then increase to the weight they can really lift. This is the process we should take as well. The muscle is amazing, you ever got up in the morning and just could not walk straight even though you did not drink at all however later you could even run. The muscle works this way, it needs to warm up and stretch before it can handle its full capacity. So when you are heading back to the gym or going for the first time go slow, warm up the muscle and gradually go up with your weights.

One more reason to warm up is to avoid injury, starting out too fast, hard, heavy can result in muscle injury and setbacks. Sometime when this happens people say it is because of age when most of the time it is due to being unreasonable when training.

Do not be afraid to set goals

If you happen to start training and feel as if you have come far, you have. Anyone who overcame foolish thinking along with other challenges and started training have certainly come far. However resolving to stay were you are because you feel this Is all you can do is not the correct way to think either. Setting realistic goals can indeed makes training enjoyable and more productive. If you are walking now then jogging and possibly running might be something realistic to shoot for. The results you seek will drastically increase as you reach each phase of your goal since each will result in a more intense form of training.

Do not get discouraged

There are challenges to training when we are not young, and it is for this reason more so we should be careful, start slow and be realistic. However the possibility of seeing changes and reaching our goals are within our reach. It may take longer because our training cannot be as intense as we would like or we may incur some setbacks from injury because of going a bit too fast or achy muscles.   Give it time and be determined to let the body get used to our the new training routine and soon we will see progress.

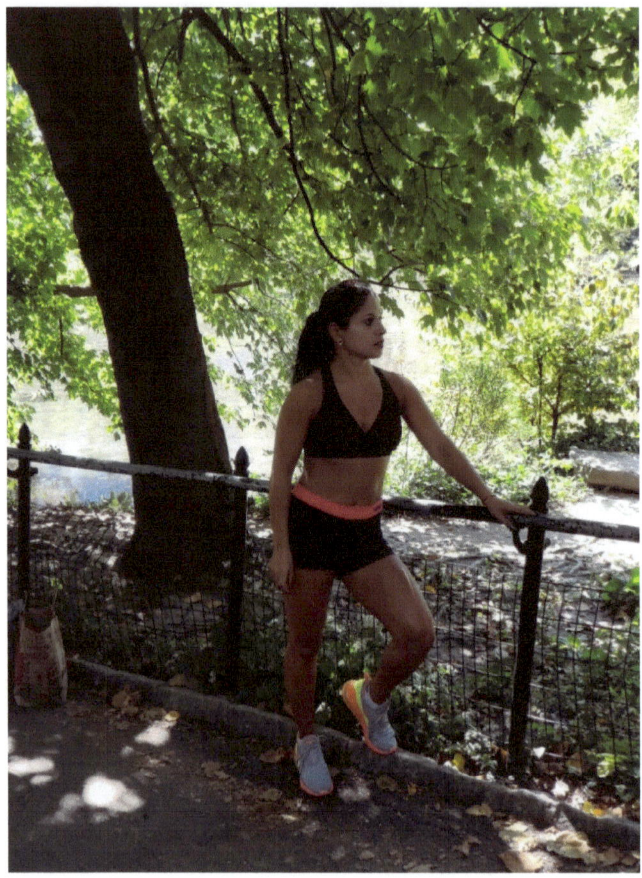

WHEN SHOULD TRAINING END?

There are so many rules people have when it comes to training. Like 'only train 45 minutes' , 'you are too old to be training'. As to our training time weather it is during our training session or our training life it really will depends on a few things, you goal, your health, your desire, you physicians instructions and you.

How Long Should Our Training Sessions Be?

A 45 minute training routine may be very good for some however, it may or may not suffice for you. If you notice that your body need more time to get results then do what you must. It is a good idea to use different machines or do different exercise for the muscle and let the muscle rest after training for a day or so. If you are following this principle then fine. However if you find your self being prone to injury during training because you are not allowing the muscle to rest 24 hours before training it again then try to do so. However as to your training sessions it self, give yourself the time to get the result you need.

Should Older People Retire from Training

I live in the United States of America, our society here seeks to retire the old as soon as possible, and I fear this philosophy has reached the gym as well. However if someone is not ill and posses the energy to train and workout then, why should they not do so? There are many people in advanced years that enjoy training, they are in great physical shape with excellent training routine. They encouraged and sometime offer tips to new people coming into the training scene. Their training keeps them in excellent physical shape while their years of training makes them indispensable as far as training knowledge and experience is concerned.

HOW FAR SHOULD WE PUSH OUR SELF

We are often amazed at what others have been able to do, it is as if we do not know our full potentials as humans. The truth is some of us never really find out our potential because we do not push our self enough. We might amaze our self of what we can do when it comes to physical training.

Of course pushing oneself does not mean straining with overly heavy weights nor injuring our self trying to do what our friend does. Pushing our self means just that - pushing OURSELF! Lets say you are running 30 minutes now for the last 3 month, how about shooting for 40 minutes this month. This is entirely possible for you because it is only 10 minutes more. Whereas if you are only doing 10 minutes runs, trying to go to 40 minutes right away might me a bit much. To push our self means trying to reach new limits, however when doing so we should do it gradually, this way we avoid injury and allow the muscle to grow.

It could be that we really have a big goal, for example to lift 200 lbs and now we are lifting 100 lbs. Although going from 100 lbs to 200 lbs can seem daunting try going up gradually by 5 lbs or even less. You can add 5 lbs each month or every 2 weeks based on how fast your body will grow. This way over time you will grow to the point of reaching 200 lbs.

We can go as far as we need to go when we do so in such a way as to allow the muscle to grow and respond.

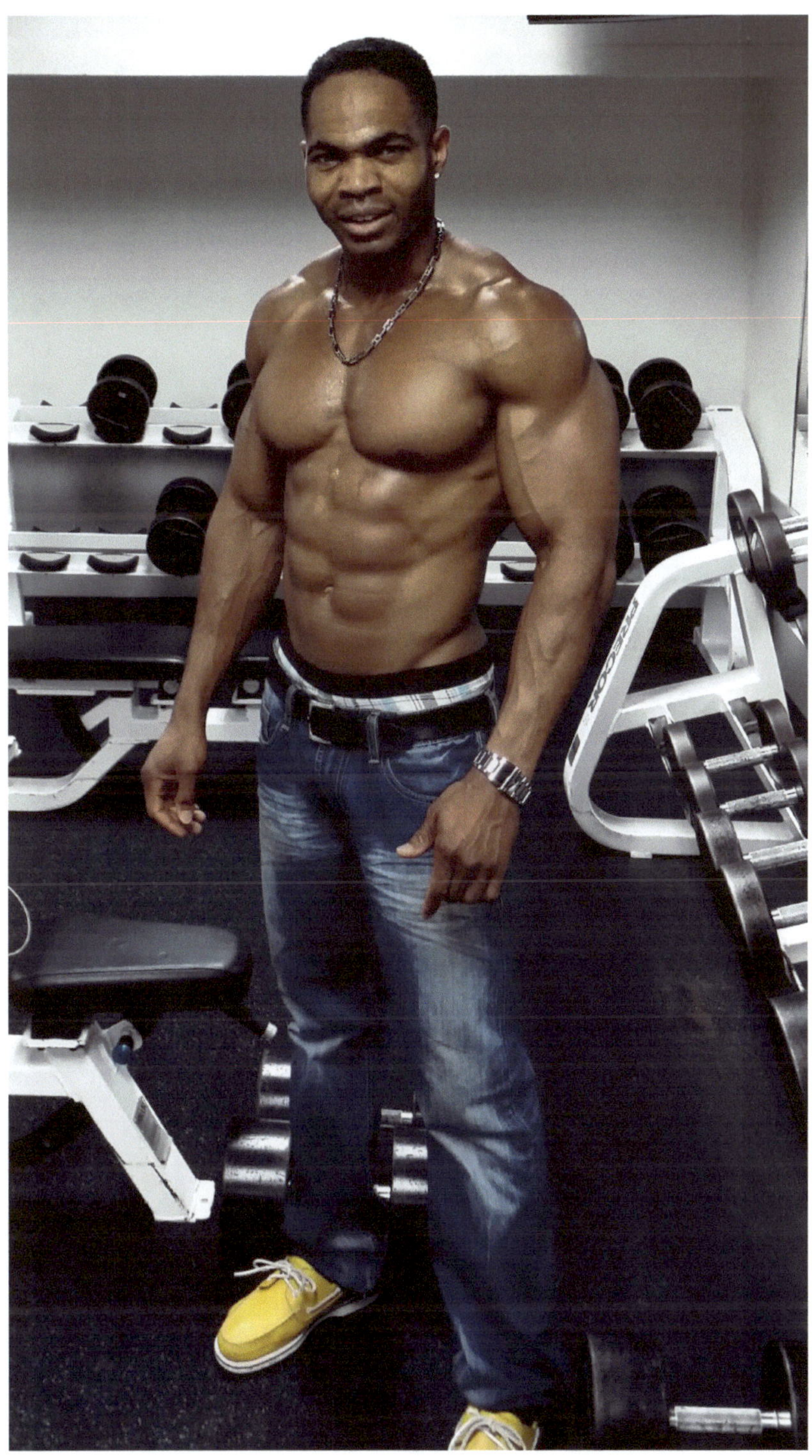

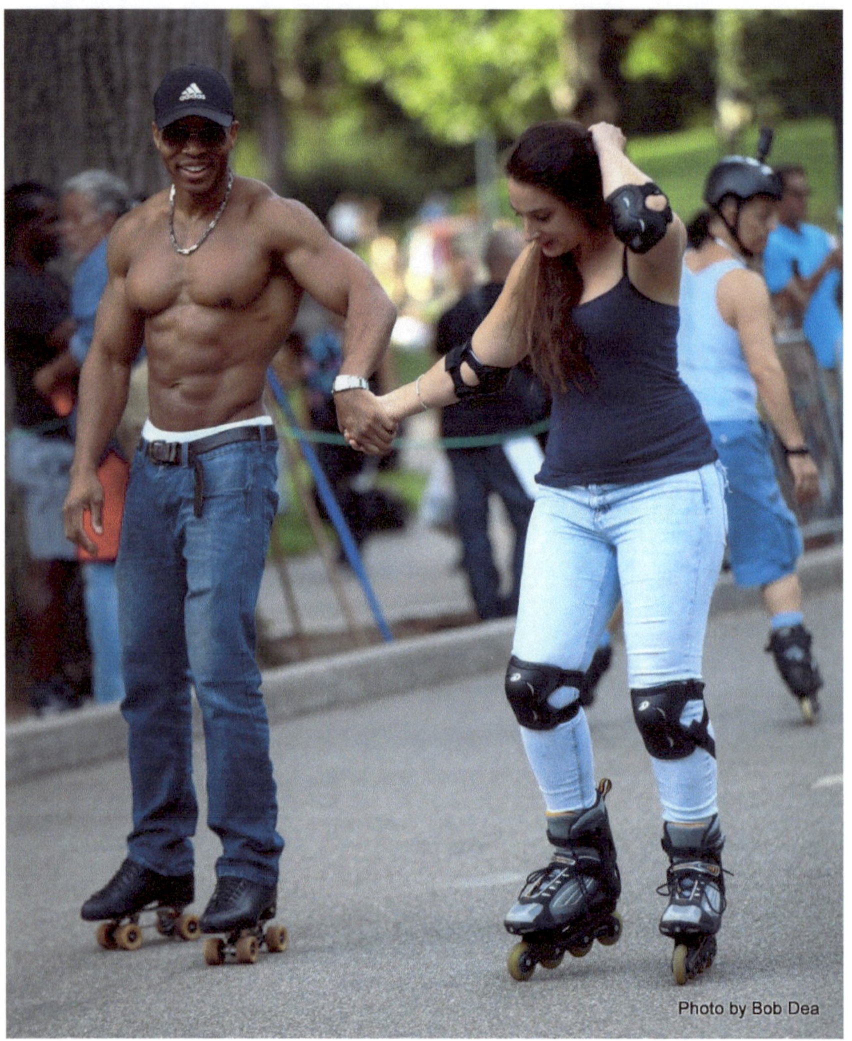

CAN EVERYONE TRAIN

Everyone can and should do some form of fitness training. Health and fitness is a core part of human life, the more healthier and fit the more easy it will be to remain mobile and avoid some illnesses.

Adjust Training with your circumstance

A relatively healthy person can perhaps run, lift weights, bike ride, doing most things that will help him/her maintain good health without issues. Someone who have not train for sometime or maybe extremely overweight or an older person or perhaps is in a wheel chair will have some training limitations. However do not lose heart, simply adjust the training to fit your needs. If running is not an options, then walking or speed walking can be very effective. If you do not have access to the gym then a local park can be a great training location. Bike riding can be replacement for some with knee problems as it offers low impact leg workout. A friend of mine who has worked our her whole life with weights cannot do so anymore so she swims, which is an excellent low impact workout.

The goal of training is to help improve our life, all of us can fine some form of training that improve our life in some way. When something does not work for you, just try something else until you find that training system that will help you reach your goals.

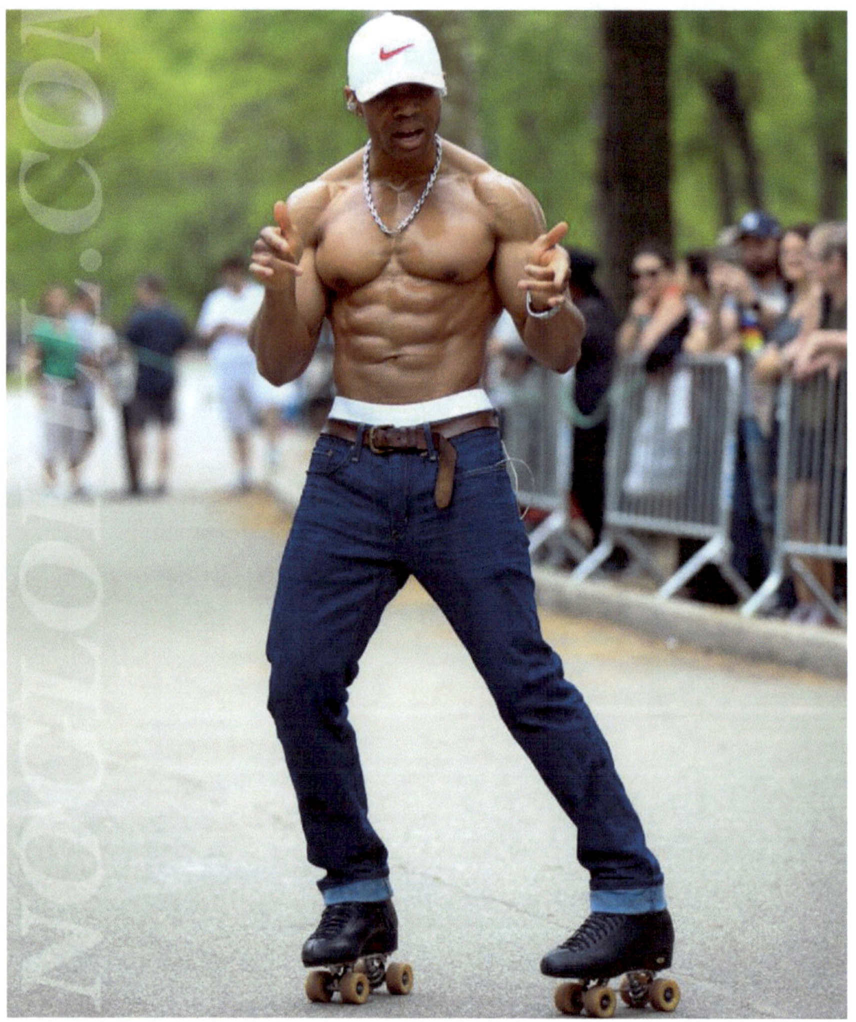

IS TRAINING EFFORT WORTH IT

There is much information and evidence to prove the benefits of a life filled with health and fitness. However as we all know - all the knowledge in the world is not enough to push someone who does not want to do something. We must all come to see or believe there is training benefits for us personally.

Find the Personal benefits

Knowing that something is good for someone else does not always drive a person to action. Most people are moved to engage in activity when there is some personal benefits to them. Lets say a father or mother always wanted to exercise and just could not find the time because of family obligation, work etc. Now after a recent Doctors visit the father is border line diabetic and has been cautioned to make some drastic changes in his life. Or perhaps the mother receives a prognoses from the doctor that her cholesterol is so high she is in danger of heart problems. Now health and fitness is not only a concerned to think about but can provide personal benefits to this family. Training is not just an option but may save their life or increase their lives, giving them more time to spend with the family they love so much. Training may also improve their life as they lose weight becoming more active and can get around better with less weight. Mentally they are also more relieved knowing that the husband or wife will be around for a few more years with the family because they took action to take care of their health and started physical training.

Because there is a personal benefits fitness training is now being done after all these years of thinking about it, now they see the value or worth of the effort to them personally.

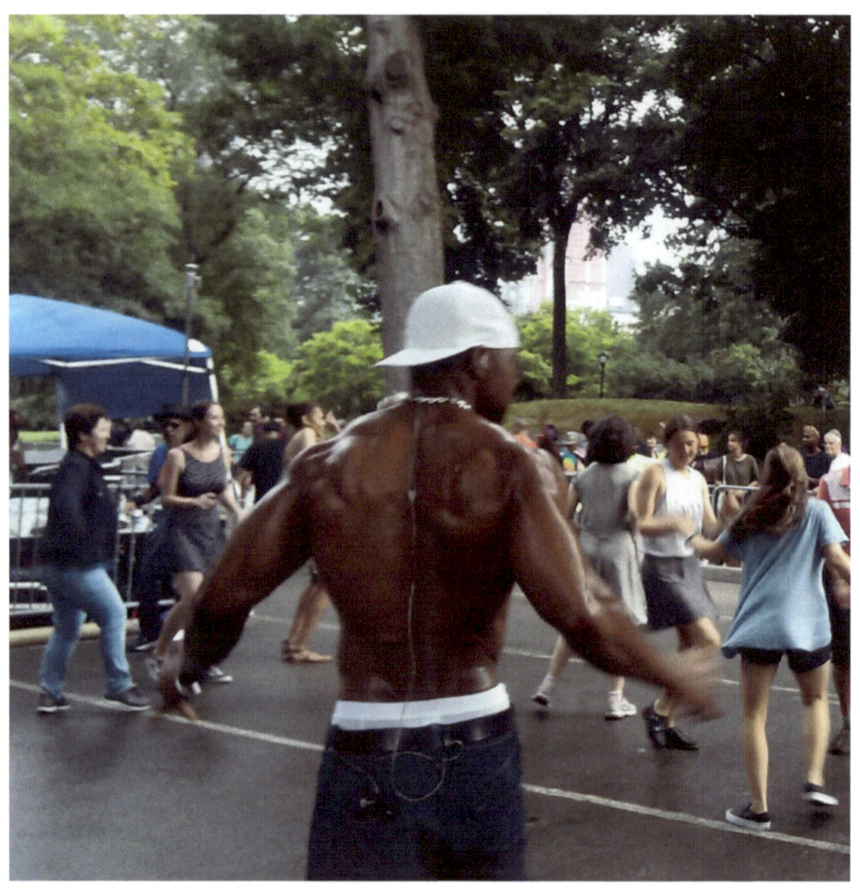

TRAINING IN THE RAIN, EXTREME HEAT OR COLD (INCLEMENT WEATHER)

What do you do when the weather is not so good for training, perhaps it is raining, snowing , freezing or too hot.   Well we train anyway despite the weather. We must be careful and take precautions though however like work that must be done despite the weather so too much our health and fitness be cared for despite the weather.

Training when it is Raining , Snowing, Too hot or too cold etc.

So the weather is crappy and you do not feel like training. What do we do now ? I am reasonable with my self and my training routine. If there is a day of torrential rainfall or unusually hot or cold weather then taking a break if fine.   However if this last for 5 or more days where by it not is effecting my training routine the it is time to think of ideas.   Drink more water, shorter runs, run indoors on treadmill within air-conditioned environment, or where is heat so as not to freeze to death, drive slower on the freezing road to the gym etc. When work must be done people think of creative ideas to get to work because we do not have a choice, so too with our training.   We should not be extremist in anything as this is not being reasonable however finding way to keep our training consistent when the weather threatens to stop us is a must.

Training is important for our health however without life we cannot train. When the weather threatens our life we should think seriously how to proceed with our training so as not to lose our life. However if the weather is not life threatening or we can find training environment that is safe during the inclement weather then we should continue training during inclement weather.

KEEP GOING EVEN WHEN TIRED

For most of us our training will take only a portion of the day, then we go on to our real life. For this reason and because effort is required to see progress we should make the best of the time we have set aside for training.

There are those moments that we must push threw when we are training, some will be physical others mental then there are both when the body and mind is screaming at you at the same time. Periodic breaks is recommended when training as this can be very helpful, however push threw the training routing even when you feel like you do now want to or are too tired to do so or are just not in the mood - lack of focus. There are many times when training that we must keep training despite how we may feel at the moment. Sometimes the brain will respond with -stop that is enough for today, you are tired and deserve a break for today! You are tires yes however this is only an excuse, do not buy it, continue to completion of your training routine even with a tried body. Training will take great physical and mental effort, it is for this very reason some people get a personal trainer or friend to keep them going.

Trainer can help us

Although a trainer can be useful for many things, keeping us going when we are tired is certainly one of them. Having someone there to push us , remind us of the reason why we are training or just give us that look can be just what is needed to continue training when tiredness kicks in.

Muscle Response takes time

Of course muscle response takes effort and to see the changes we dream of will take more time than we are sometime willing to put in. For this reason than we most keep going even when we feel tired because this is what will give us the results we seek. When we can push beyond what we feel or think we can do we put our self in another place where we were not before - we can now possible burn more calories or build bugger muscles because we have reached another level in our training. In time if we keep fighting we may even surpass this level, becoming more consistent thus seeing even better results.

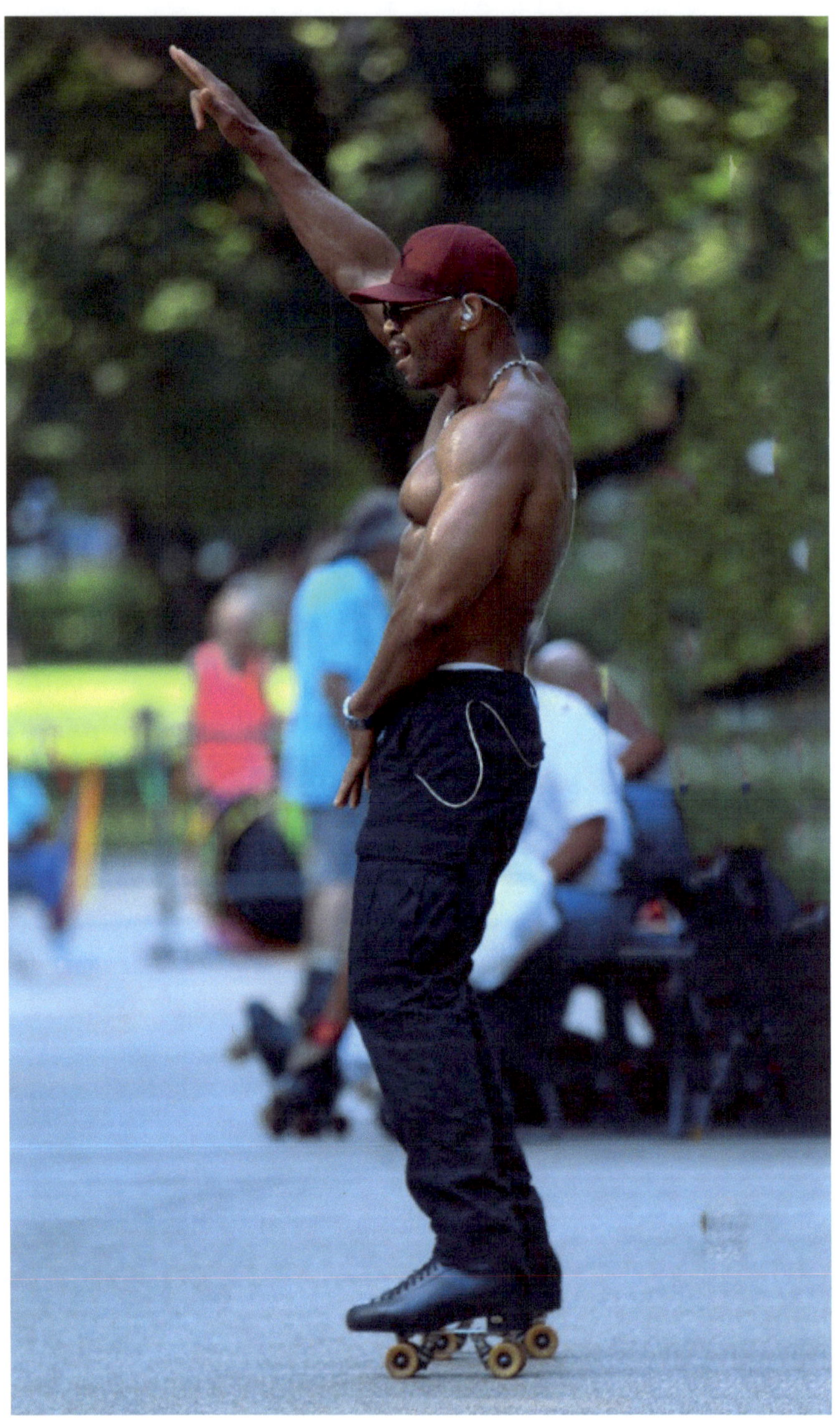

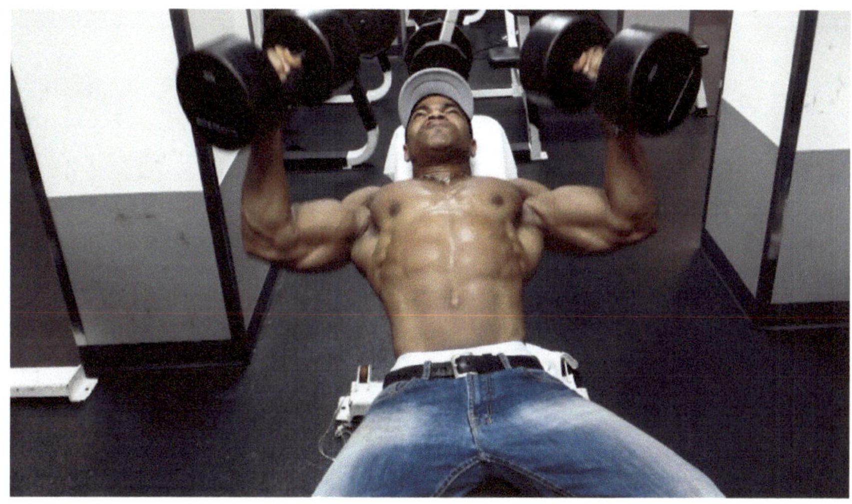

THE RIGHT AND WRONGS OF TRAINING

Do not be too strict when it comes to fitness training, and do not drive yourself and other people crazy with rules. Remember health and fitness is about you, improving your life so as to make you happy.

Enjoy training

Fitness training should be enjoyable not a chore to get done with as soon as possible. Training is something we want to be able to do for years to come not a summer goal. For this to happen it has to be enjoyable, something we like to do and can do. Too many people have all these do's and don't about training that sometime it is daunting just to think about it. From how long we should train to how many sets or reps and when and how each sets and reps should be done. The rules just never seems to end. Do yourself a favor and enjoy your training with or without all those rules. Do you like 2 sets, then do 2 sets. Do you like to train at midnight, then train at midnight. Do you like to training for 10 hours then train for 10 hours. Training is your right so do not let anyone make it wrong for you. There are training basics of to follow like warming up, not lifting too heavy, proper motion and posture to avoid injury. however once you have these basic training rules down then go train your heart out.

There is a place for rules and commands, however adding too much rules to your training can be annoying, taking the fun our of training. When things do not go as planned just adjust and keep going. If schedule shift take it with a grain of salt, smile and adjust. Keep your training interesting and fun.

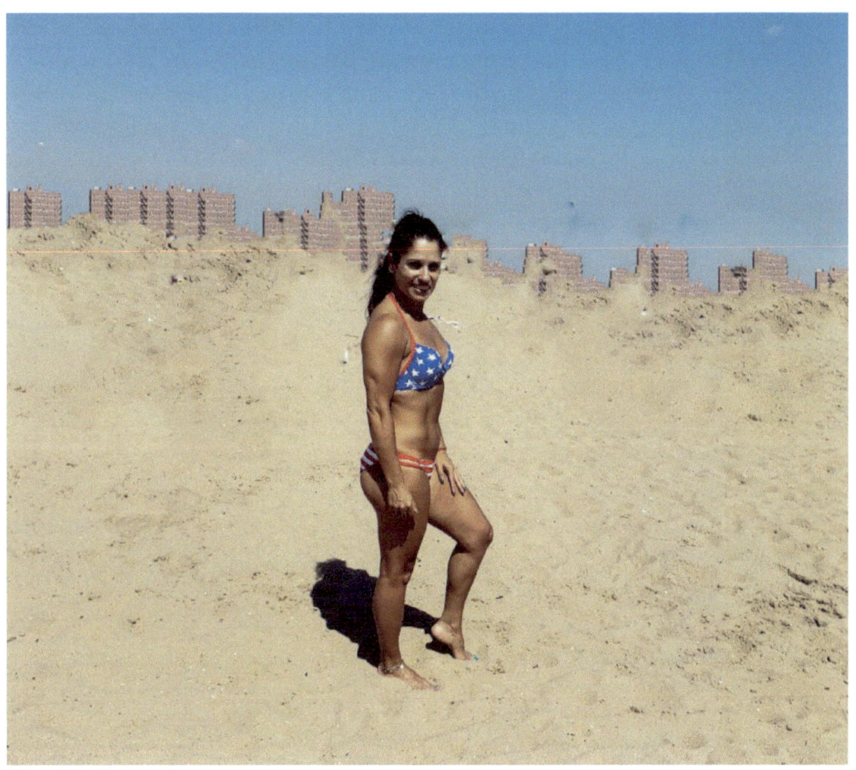

THE SACRIFICES WE MAKE TO TRAIN

Getting up early to train before work, training after work or during work or on the weekends. We make so much effort to stay healthy and fit.

Seen & Unseen Sacrifices to train

Sometime training requires sacrifice that goes unnoticed even by ourselves. We may go to sleep early to get needed rest so as to have energy to train to the disappointment of friends who would like to hang our like old times.   Perhaps those old times had other high cost that came along with them that we do not mind forgetting like falling asleep at work the next day, falling asleep at the wheel driving to work or being a mindless dummy when we try to be a support to our wife and children the day after.   Our diet choices revolve around our fitness training, choosing salad or grilled chicken rather than tasty fried chicken may be a better choice to support our training routine.   After a friend of mine died of Diabetes I realize the seriousness of taking care of my health with a good diet. I have never found a person that regrets eating better whether by choice or because their training routing forced them to do so. There are times when our training my requires lower alcoholic intake or no alcoholic beverages at all which can really put a dampening on the our night life. You and I both know that less alcohol in our life can means less trouble, some of us are still paying the price of a little too much alcohol years ago. Being forced to stop or lower our intake is not usually a thing I hear people complaining about, most celebrate it. Personally I train when I am on vacation to the surprise of my friends who prefer to be on vacation when on vacation without any form of training. However I find the sacrifice of training on vacation to be well worth it since I do not fall so far behind when I return to civilization back home. Another sacrifice that may go unnoticed is our determination to think positive with motivating thought so as to keep our self and others going. I find most of the people in the gym very positive about training and extremely encouraging, not a mental resolve that comes easy to humans. It takes effort to be positive to yourself and others each day however this we do to encourage our self and others not to give up with obvious benefits. We are more of a delight to be around and we are our own mental life coach for the most part.

A life of health and fitness will without fail require sacrifices, some we are aware and others we may not realize however the benefits will far out weigh the sacrifice we put forth.

IS TRAINING PHYSICAL OR MENTAL

Perhaps this is a strange question for many since physical fitness obviously uses our muscles without which training is not possible.

Physical & Mental

Although Training does require the use of our muscles thus making it physical in nature try as you might to get a mentally discouraged or mentally depressed person to go out with you to do some fun exercise. Try yourself to go out when you are not 'mentally' in the mood to go out and do some physical exercise. You see although fitness is physical in nature, without the right mood which is mental in nature, we will not train.

Being ready and available to train is half the battle, we then need to be mentally prepared to carry our out training. The right mental attitude toward health and fitness build desire to train without which we will find something more important to do with our time. As important as it is to be physically ready so too it is important to be mentally ready to train. Some would argue that being mentally ready to train is even more important than being physically ready as can be seen from the turnout at any gym. It is not always the physically fit that comes to train but mothers, fathers, overweight individuals, sick individuals , wheel chair individuals etc. When you find your self having difficulty training and you are not injured or bed ridden, It is time to take steps to address our mental training resolve.

We must keep our self mentally ready, determined and encouraged when it comes to fitness training because then we will make the necessary steps to train.

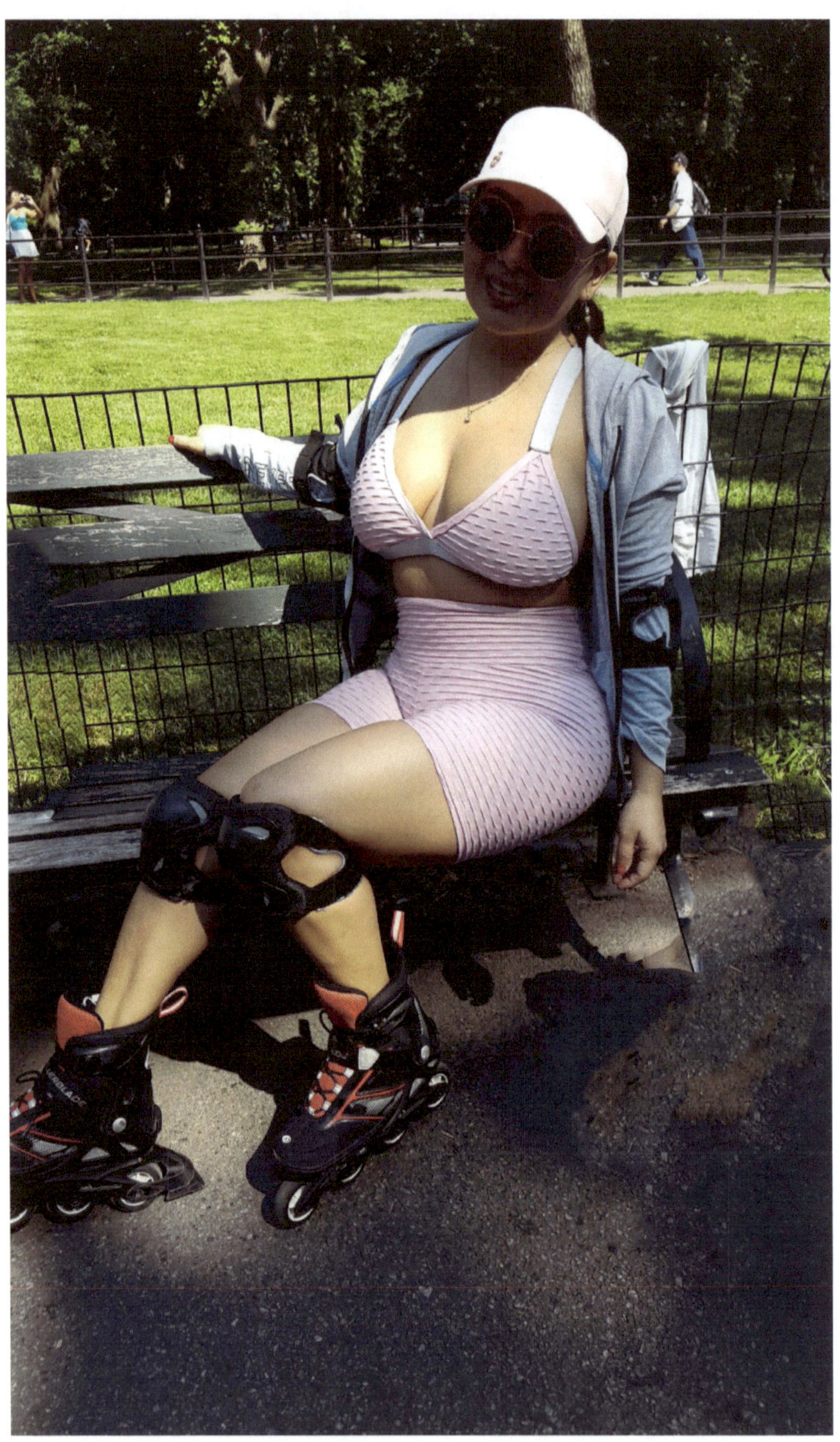

HEALTH AND FITNESS IS ALWAYS CHANGING

We are creatures of habits and many times reject changes. However a life of fitness is fraught with changes.   As we learn new ways to benefit the body we adapt, as we become more experiences at training over the years we develop new routines and new ways to do the same things in less time.

Health and fitness is progressive, as we grow muscles become stronger forcing us to adapt or change our training routine.   A new training routine will produce further growth in physical strength that will then move us to make more changes to our training routine. This is not a life of stagnation except wherein such involve a regular training schedule or the same training location. Aside from these two things our training life is one of growth and change. Muscle growth and change along with mental growth and change as our training learning curve expands. I have made so many combination of training routines over the years and I am still creating new training routines.

Growth will not end as long was we continue to train, and as long as we continue to grow we will continue to change.

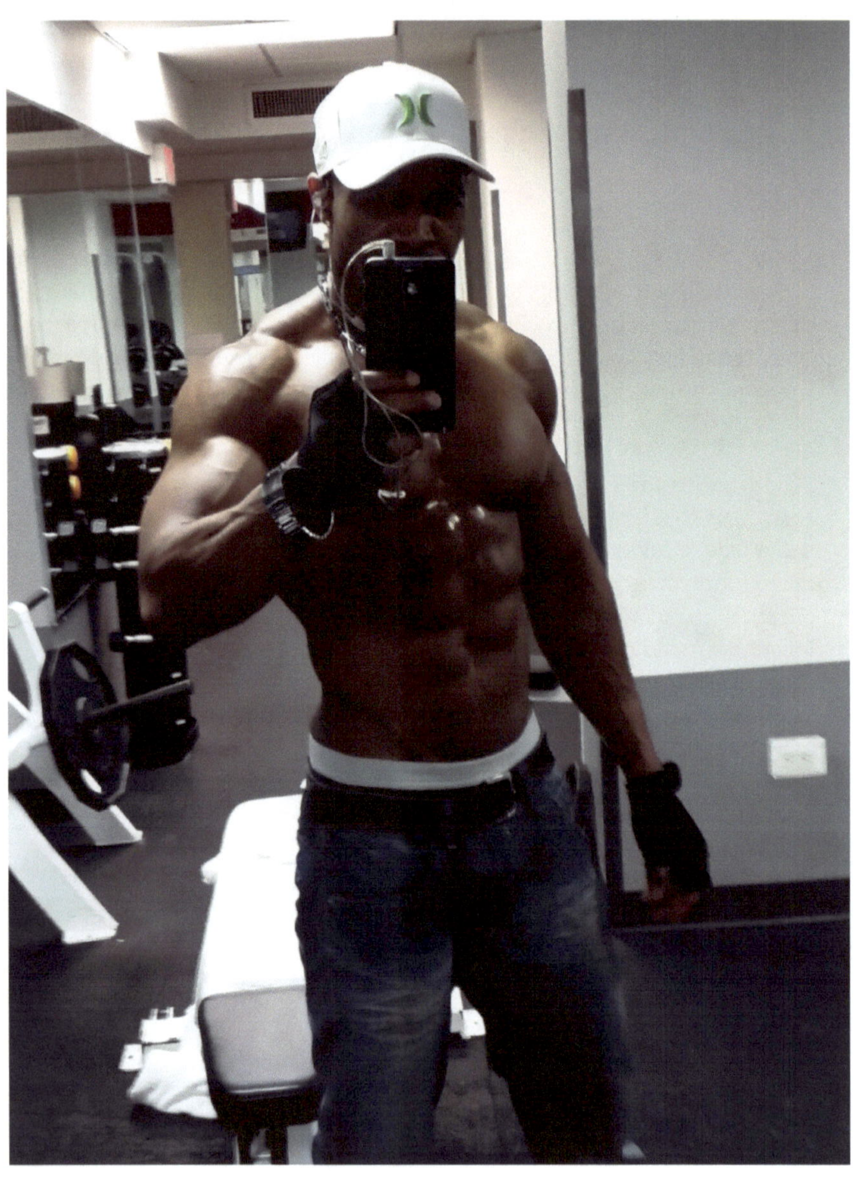

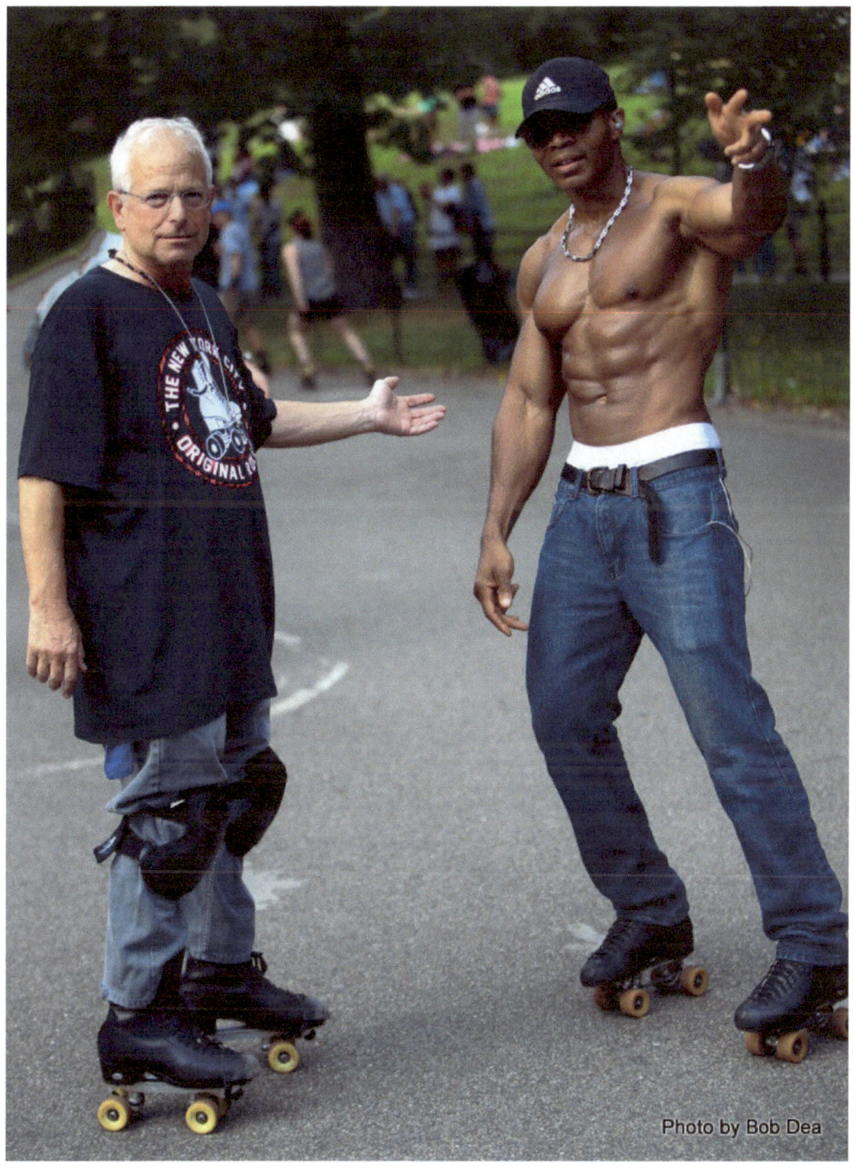

THE POWER OF BEING POSITIVE

Without question a positive mental attitude has been know to foster success
in almost every walk of life, health and fitness is no exception. Being

positive when it comes to health and fitness is probably one of the most important thing aside from training itself.

When we a positive we tend to look at the bright side or the half filled glass of a life of training rather than the bad side or half empty glass of training. We can see small changes as a means to push forward rather than becoming discourage at just such a little change. The positive person is a source of encouragement and motivation for everyone as they make training fun, easy and a joy to look forward to. Even injury is looked at differently by a positive person as they try to see what can be learned or how they can continue to train with the uninjured parts of their body or even be an encouragement to others that are not injured. I remember an Olympic athlete that injured herself with a broken leg then went to encourage her team mates by chairing them on through the rest of the games rather than sulking or staying home by herself complaining about her injury. She was happier and even her teammates was motivated to have her continued support.

Although anger and frustration or even depression push one to train those who continue to train do so because of a positive mental outlook on life and their health. Further more training places are usually filled with positive people encouraging us to set and reach new goals. I once heard the story of a man who is always at the gym but never training just talking to people, seems he knows where find positive encouraging people to be around.

EVERYONE WANT TO BE HEALTHY

The good thing about a life of health and fitness is that everyone wants to be healthy so we do not have to feel wired telling people about our fitness routine or fitness goal, even when such comes between some important events.

Unlike other hobbies that people cannot nor do not with to understand, health and fitness is universal so explaining to someone that we cannot stay up late or socialize because of prior fitness commitments is not a difficult thing. Most people will even commend us to now that we are making such effort to care for hour health.   This along with the fact that most people envy those who chose a life of health and fitness is great motivation to continue. Sometime we can even become the reason why some return to training. I once had someone confess to me that he was motivated to return to training as a result of seeing me train. Training is so universal that even young people love to exercise and train. I remember shopping in for some vegetables next to a mother and child, the mother said to the little girl who was just steering my muscles - 'his muscles are because he eats these vegetables honey'. I was encouraged to know that even in such a little thing I could help encourage someone to eat more healthier.

There are few places you will go where people frown on you for choosing a life of fitness and health, even more so, there are few people who would not look up to you for choosing a life of fitness and health.   Rest assure you will not go wrong with a life of fitness and health further more it may surprise you to find that there are more support for such a life that you might have imagined and from people that you might not have thought. When a local over weigh man stopped to talk with me and encouraged me by stating how he wishes to get back in shape, I realize that he was not happy with his condition, I had motivated him to reconsider his training. It was unexpected because I sometime feel that people are happy with their life even when they have a few extra pounds, however I was very happy to know that I encouraged him some.

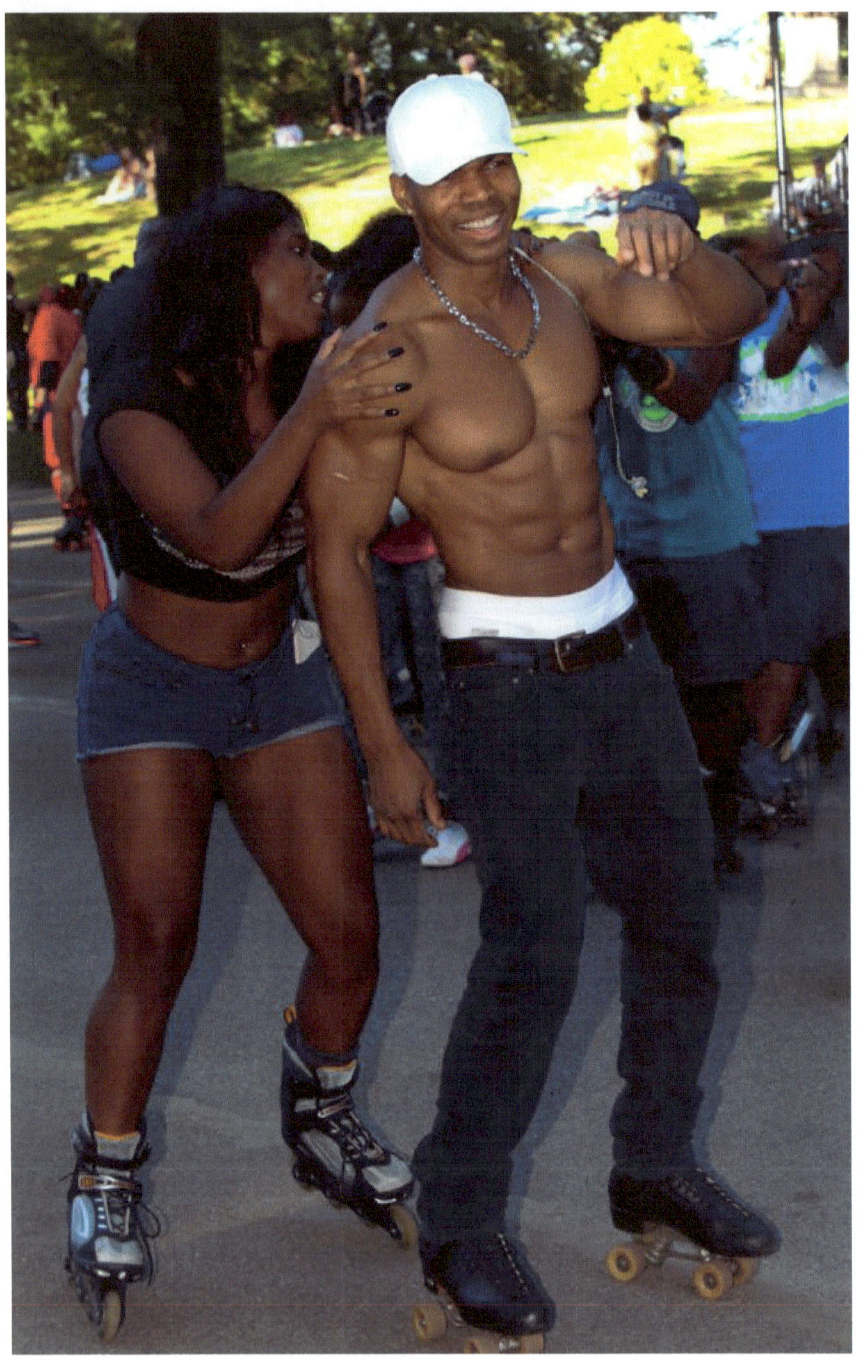

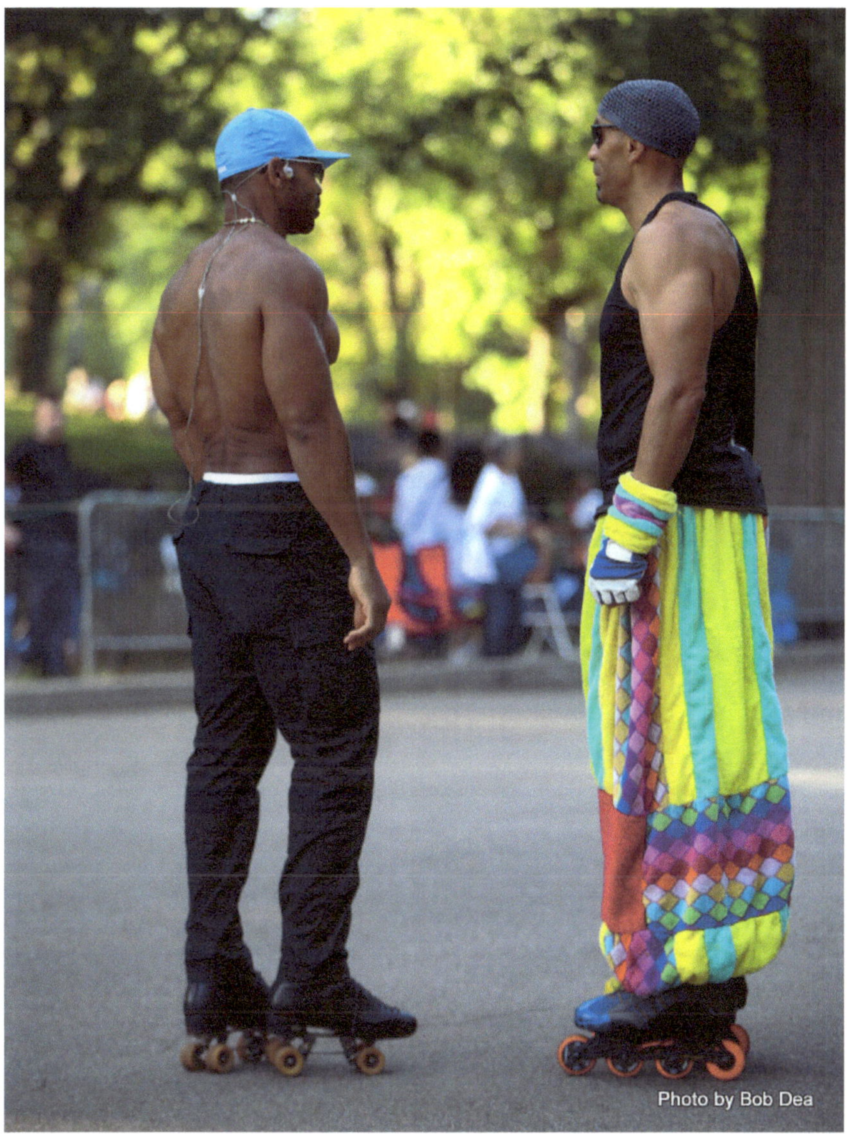

WHEN WE DON'T KNOW WHAT TO DO

There is nothing worst than a lost soul in this world and when it comes to training this applies even more so since there is unending mounds of training information we can get lost in, not to mention the hundreds of 'experts' ready to lead us astray for a dollar or even free.

A Good Example

One principle I like to follow when it comes to learning a new field is follow those who can lead by example. Even if I know nothing about the new field, one who have made a success of it should know what they are talking about, so too with training. Look at the person providing the instructions to see if he or she is a good example, are in shape? Do they have muscles? Are they over weight? Have they been help someone else lose weight? Have they been able to help someone else gain muscles?

If the one training or providing training instructions is an example themselves or have training examples in other people they have helped then you know you are going in the right direction. Safe to say that if they can make their training work for them self and other then that training can work for you as well. Once we can select a trustworthy trainer the next step is to train, fitness knowledge is of no value unless we can put it to good use in our lives. The next step would be to continue on a training routine until we have arrived at our goal.

So don't be afraid to start training event if you do not know what to do. Look for a good trainer example, someone who themselves have demonstrated over time that they know how to make their training technique work in themselves or others. Then follow through with your training by having a good training routine each week.

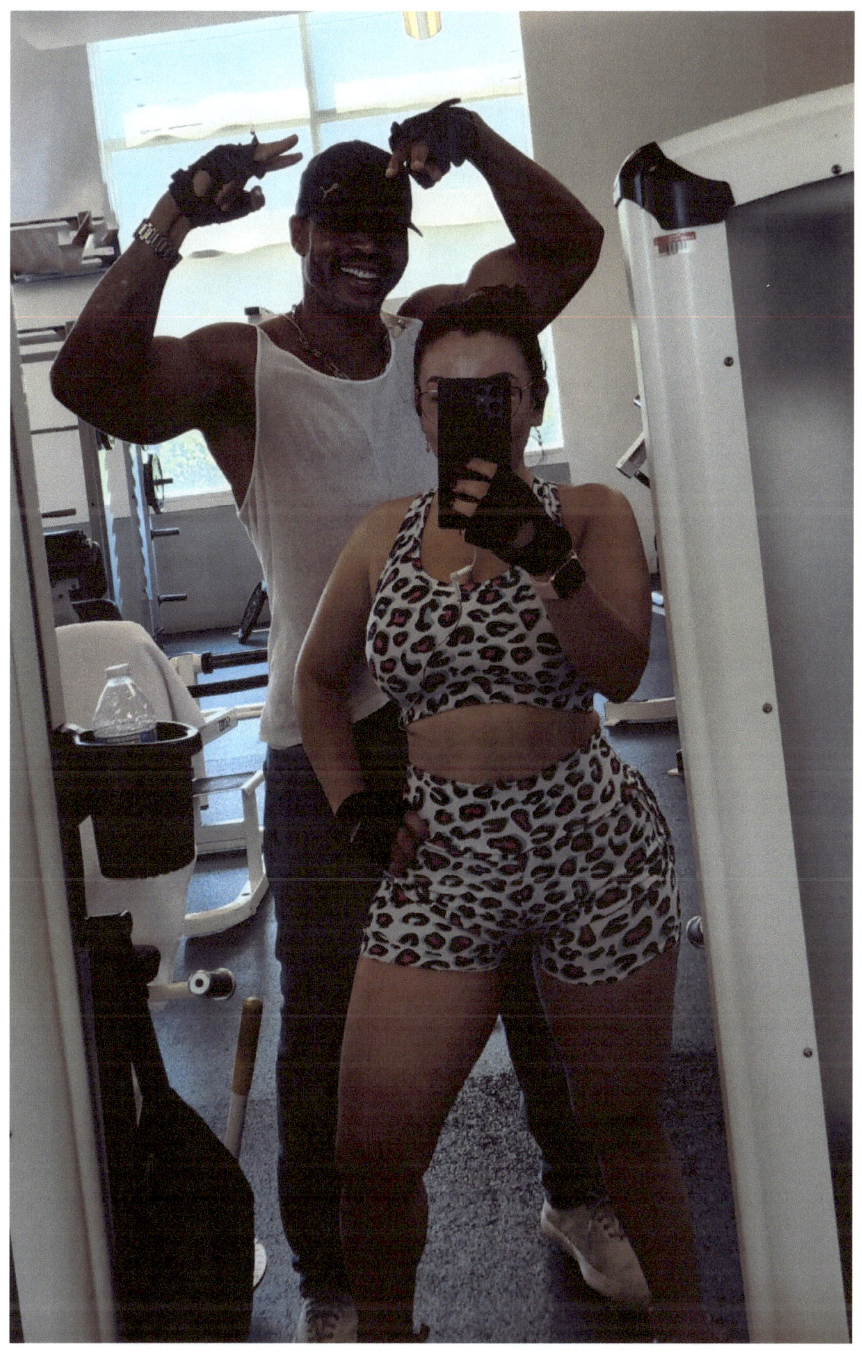

THE IMPORTANT THINGS IN LIFE

The ability to prioritize or remember the important things in life will help us succeed, especially since our time is limited. Health and fitness is certainly on the top of the list of important things in life since the longevity or quality of life can be increased but being healthy and having a good fitness routine.

Longevity or quality of life

To most people one of the most important thing is longevity or quality of life that they have to live. Living life to the fullest has always been a concern for humans and they have been willing to do almost anything to make that this possible. Sickness and bad health can greatly decrease the length and quality of our life however health and fitness can extend our life and even increase the quality of our life.

What price can we then put on longevity or an increased quality of life. Certainly fitness and health should be on the top of the important things in our life since it can be instruments in increasing the length and quality of our life. To this end we may have to neglect some things or remove or decrease some time wasters so as to have time for fitness and health. The strange thing about important things of life is that we do not always make them important. How many people are overweight for no apparent reason? How many people pay gym membership and do not go? How many people you know personally that have sickness that can be reversed or healed by a lifestyle change but refuse to make the change? Though health and fitness is important for many, it is still a challenge to make it one of the important thing in our life even when our life is threatened and we know a healthy fitness routine can help. Longevity and quality of life unfortunately is sometime not enough by itself to make us put health and fitness as one of the important things in our life.

Priorities

Set aside time to do the important things in life and neglect the things that are not as important. Without proper time management we can waste important time on things that are not important in life, leaving us with little or no time for the important things like health and fitness. Since the very life we live can be extended or its quality increased or decreased we need to think seriously about putting time aside for fitness and health. It may be that we have to set a schedule for our self to follow or a routine or even reminders to stick to our fitness and health routine. Even then we must fight to stick to our schedule since as anyone knows there is always sometime trying to get in the way of a schedule. However since health and fitness effect the quality and even length of our life we must do everything possible to stick to our health and fitness routine.

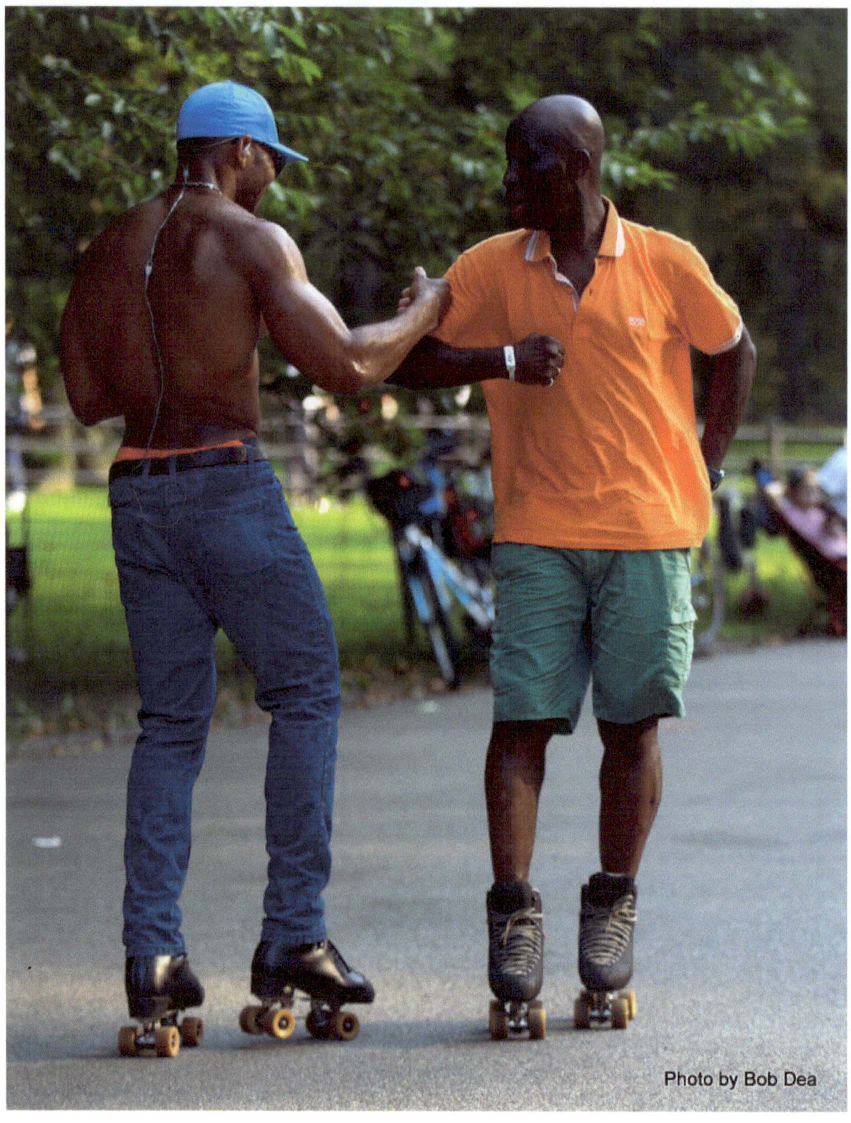

HEALTHY COMPETITION HELPS MOTIVATE TRAINING

Our training is for our benefit, to improve our health and life. For this reason we should not discourage our self by comparing our results with others. Although comparing our self or our routine with others can be negative and cause us to lose sight of our progress and training results. A healthy competition with our self or friends to finish or reach a new goal can be encouraging, adding life to our training.

Running a marathon with friends for example can be fun as you each try to see if reaching the end is possible or even who can get their first. Fitness training in the gym can also be more lively when we try to reach new goals among our friends by lifting heavier or increasing our sets or repetitions. These fun competition can help us push our self and reach new fitness goals with fond memories.

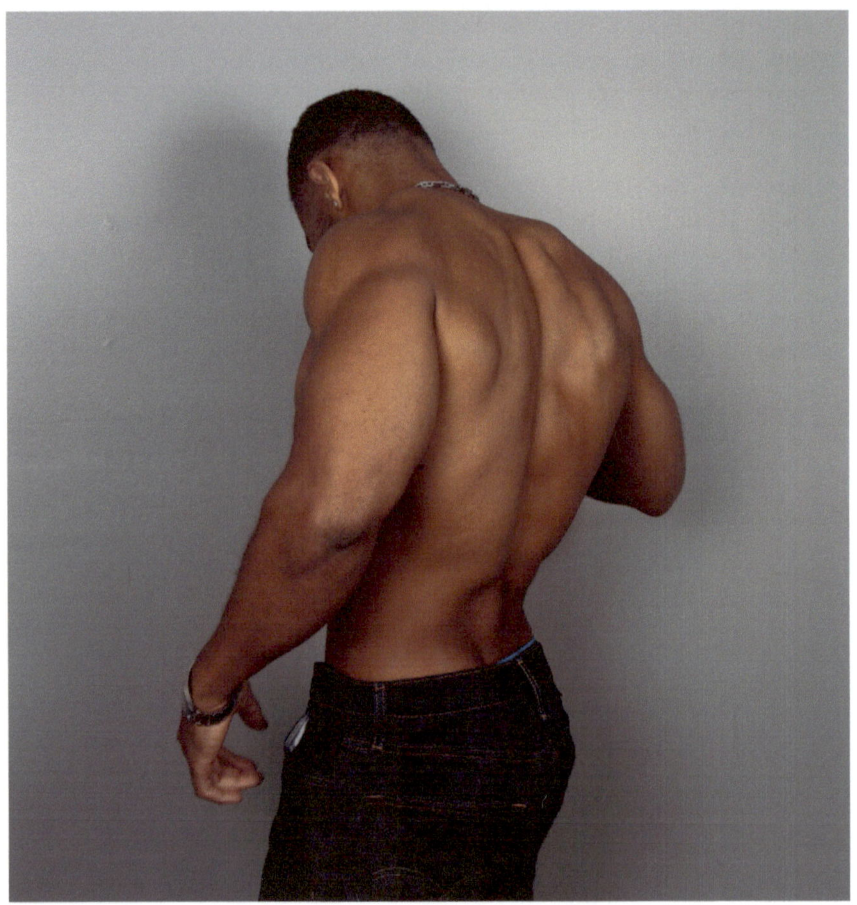

IS SOMETHING WRONG WITH OUR TRAINING

Sometime we need to make a change or adjustment to our training. How do we know when something is wrong with our training routine.   Good question since training styles can be different since training is designed to accomplish different things

Training that does Not accomplishing its purpose for you

There are roads all over the world and most are fine to walk or drive on, however when the road does not get us to our destination then it is the wrong road. So too with our training, Although the training may not in itself be wrong, if it is not designed to get us to our goal then it is not the training for us and need to be changed. Find the training that will help you reach your goal then your training will be right for you. An example would be someone trying to build muscles, running the marathon might not be the training routing for them at this time no matter how noble that may seem. A more ideal training might be a gym routine filled with isolation body parts workout for an hour or two a few times a week.

Training that is No Good

There are some roads that are just no good and lead to no where but death if we walk or drive on them. So too some training will serve no purpose for no one. If you have such a training routine then stop immediately and change it. Training routing involving life risking exercises designed to be different or get 'views' should be illuminated from your training routine immediately. Health and fitness should improve our life not put our life in danger.

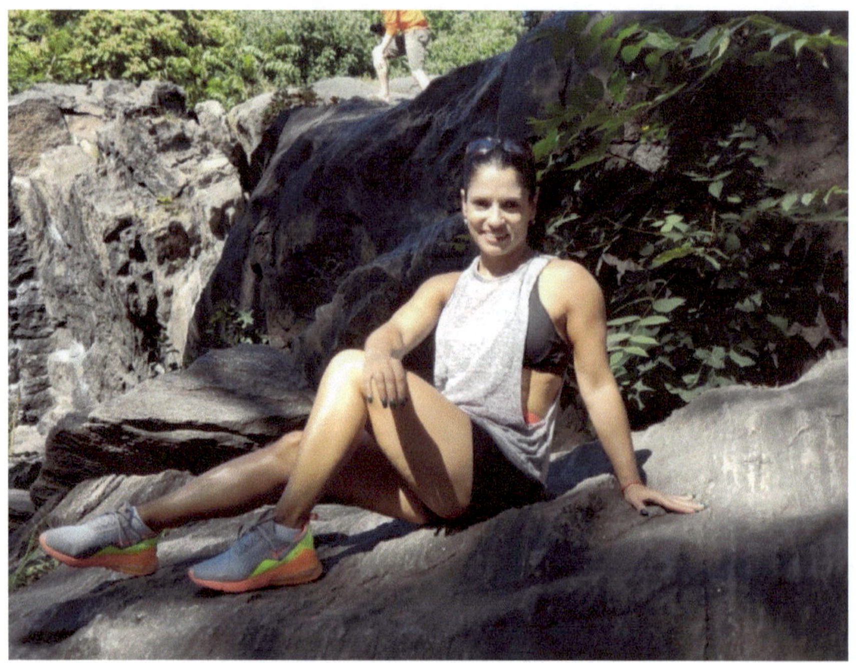

TRAINING HILLS HELP US AVOID TRAINING MONOTONY

One of the benefits of change is that it helps us avoid monotony or boredom. Sometime we complain when things change, because when we get used to things we can have a hard time changing. Another reason why change is frustrating is because it makes things a bit harder especially since we were so used to the old way

There are times when change is thrown upon us and other times when we seek out or make needed changes because we feel a need even though such change may or may not be a bit difficult to get used to. Fitness monotony can be avoided if we make periodic changes to our training routine and even to our training schedule. Lets say we always start our training with the treadmill walk, we can change it up for a few weeks by starting with the stair master, at first it may feel very different or even a bit more difficult walking up the hills instead of on a flat surface. however with a little time we will get use to it and possible learn to love walking up the stairs first thing instead of just walking on the treadmill. Or perhaps our training includes cardio for the past year with some weight training, to push our self a bit we can include swimming for the next moth or two, this will certainly change things up a bit. Yes swimming is a bit difficult if we have not been doing it for some time, however the benefits can be amazing. Or Adding Group training to our fitness routine, this might require some people skills depending on the training group, however the challenge of learning how to workout or train with a group will certainly add some laughter and fun to the your training routine and possibly some light competition.

The hills or challenges that makes our training a bit more difficult at times will also help us avoid a monotonous training life.

ACTION SPEAKS LOUDER THAN WORDS

Fitness is about doing, no amount of knowledge meditative thinking bring us to our fitness goal without action.   There are some who know much about Health and fitness and other who speak even more. I have listen to some amazing conversation by fitness experts or those who are in the know where fitness is concerned. However in the end Health and fitness is truly simple, those who are willing to train and take care of their health will be successful whereas those who are unwilling to train or take care of their health will not.

With basic knowledge of fitness coupled with a training routing we can begin to see and feel changes in a short time. I am not against gaining more knowledge and becoming an expert in the field of health and fitness, this is a great thing. The more we know about out field the better we will do and success can be even more evident. However even with more knowledge the basics of health and fitness will apply , we will only be healthier or fit when we apply what we learn. We must exercise, we must eat well, we must rest and we must maintain a healthy training routine. Someone looks great because they train, the result follows the action of doing what must be done to look and feel healthy.

So if we must speak about training lets do so after or during the training sessions and lets at least have result to show from hours of training, then others will take our words even more seriously.

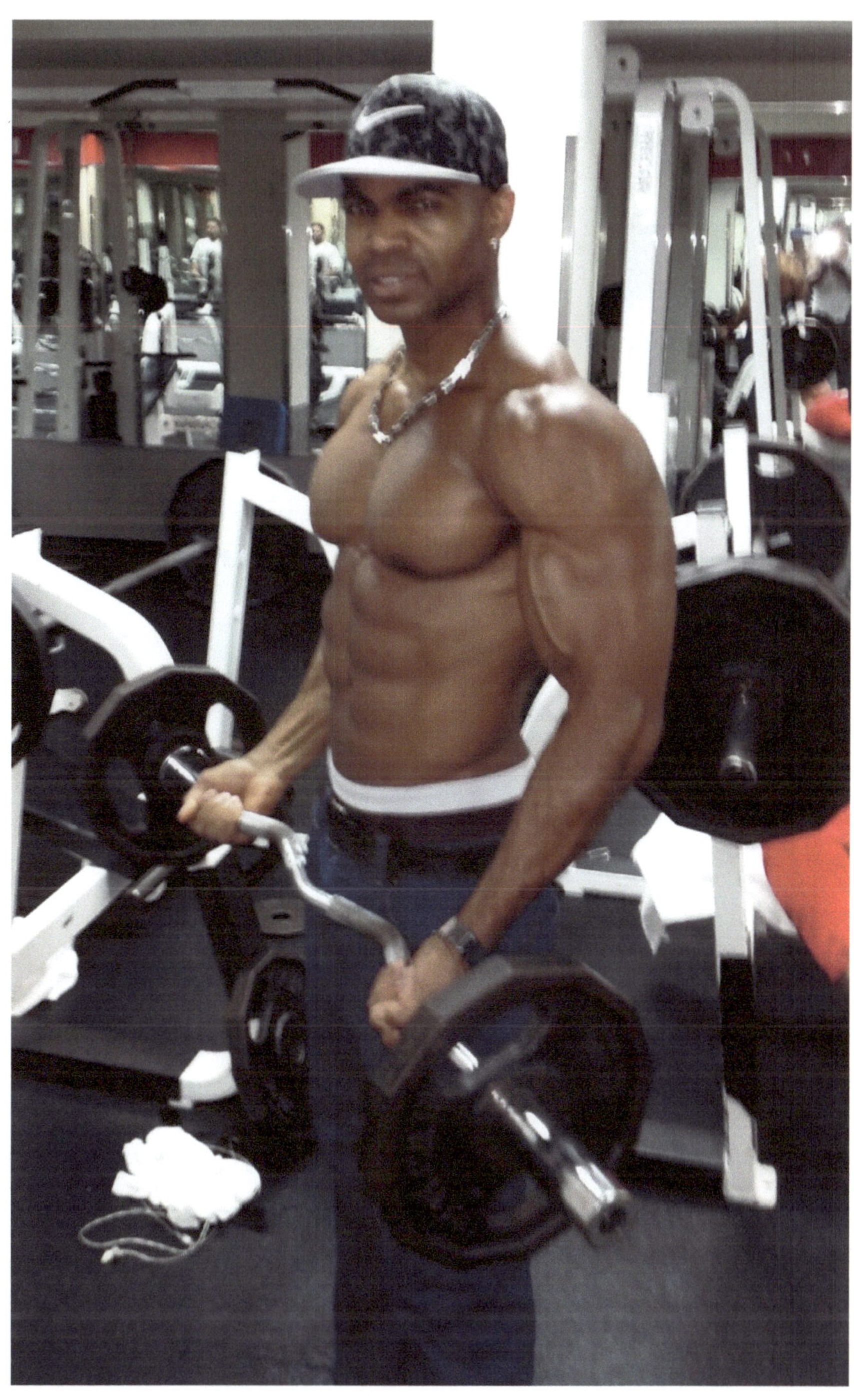

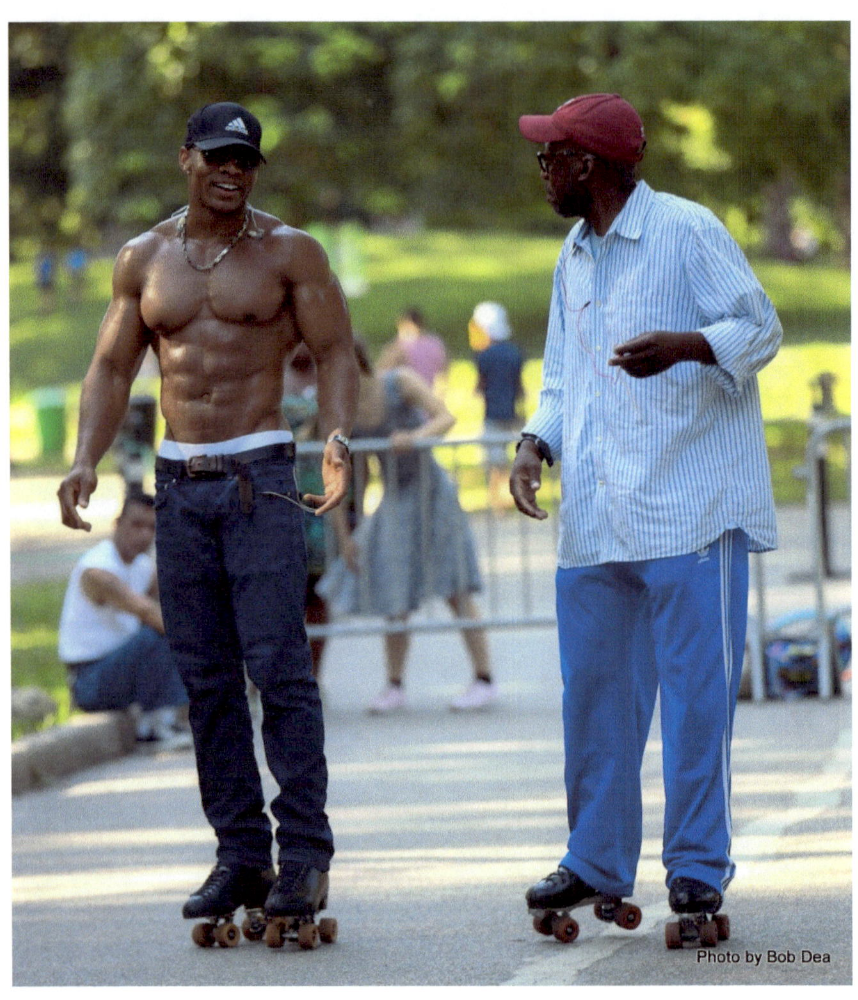
Photo by Bob Dea

ABOUT THE AUTHOR

Training has always been a love of my life. Some time over the years I train for hours. I love to learn new training techniques and push my self to new limits. I have always looked for different ways to motivate me and keep me training over the years as I have come to realize that training is as much mental as it is physical.

https://noglokel.com

Training Videos